Copyright

All rights reserved. No part of this publication maybe reproduced, distributed, or transmitted in any form or by any means, including photocopying, recording, or other electronic or mechanical methods, without the prior written permission of the publisher, except in the case of brief quotations embodied in critical reviews and certain other noncommercial uses permitted by copyright law.

Contents

What Is Inflammatory bowel disease (IBD) 6

Types of IBD 7

Comparing IBD and IBS 9

Causes and risk factors 11

Symptoms 14

Complications 15

Diagnosis 16

Treatment 18

IBD Diet 20

What's in an IBD diet plan? 21

What foods reduce inflammation and other symptoms of IBD? 24

Foods to Avoid with IBD 27

What to Eat During a Crohn's or Colitis Flare ... 28

IBD DIET RECIPES 30

Crayfish salad with rice 30

Broccoli & kale green soup 32

Bouillabaisse 34

Roasted root vegetable soup 37

Blueberry protein smoothie bowl 40

Quick no-tomato sauce 42

Chicken salad with sweet potato mash 45

Prawn and chorizo paella 47

Coronation chicken with rice 50

Gluten free tabbouleh 54

Courgetti 56

Fish or veggie cakes 57

Leeks, sprouts and broccoli with lemon herb sauce 60

Easy chicken basquaise 62

Sweet potato chips 67

Lemon cake bars 68

High protein breakfast pancakes 72

Smoked salmon frittata 74

Milk kefir recipe 77

Swede chips 80

Easy Japanese 'sushi' handrolls 82

Beef or veggie lentil dhal 84

Lemongrass steamed sea bass 89

Nightshade free guacamole 93

Zesty summer salad 94

Chicken wrapped in bacon with pineapple and roasted vegetables 96

Gluten free teriyaki sauce 99

Bacon, eggs and avocado 101

Gluten free teriyaki sauce 102

Egg fried rice 104

Easy chicken basquaise 107

Turkey and spinach meatball 111

What Is Inflammatory bowel disease (IBD)

Inflammatory bowel disease (IBD) refers to several long-term conditions that involve inflammation of the digestive tract, or gut.

It is estimated that about 3.1 million Americans suffer from IBD. Males and females are affected equally. Ulcerative colitis and Crohn's disease may occur at any age, including young children but occur most often in young adults. Most cases of Ulcerative colitis and Crohn's disease are diagnosed before age 30. Crohn's disease tends to occur in families and in certain ethnic groups, such as Eastern European Jews. About 5 percent to 8 percent of patients may have a family member with IBD and about 20 percent to 25 percent of patients may have a close relative with the condition. However, it can occur in any ethnic group and in members of families where no one else has these diseases.

Types of IBD

The two main types of IBD are ulcerative colitis and Crohn's disease.

Ulcerative colitis

This condition causes inflammation in the large intestine, or colon. There are several different classes of ulcerative colitis, depending on location and severity. These are:

- Ulcerative proctitis: This type occurs when inflammation stays within the rectum. It tends to be the mildest form of ulcerative colitis.

- Universal colitis, or pancolitis: This type occurs when inflammation spreads across the entire colon.

- Proctosigmoiditis: The type occurs when the rectum and lower end of the colon experience inflammation.

- Distal colitis: This type occurs when inflammation extends from the rectum and up the left colon.

- Acute severe ulcerative colitis: This is a rare type that causes inflammation across the entire colon, leading to severe symptoms and pain.

Crohn's disease

Crohn's disease can affect any part of the digestive tract between the mouth and the anus.

However, it most commonly develops in the final section of the small intestine and colon.

This type of IBD has become more common over time. In fact, around 500,000 people in United States now have it, according to the National Institute of Diabetes and Digestive and Kidney Diseases (NIDDK).

They also suggest that Crohn's disease is most likely to develop when a person is aged 20–29.

Comparing IBD and IBS

There are some similarities between IBS and IBD. For example, they can both lead to changing bowel habits and pain in the abdomen. The symptoms of both also tend to flare-up for short periods, then go into remission.

Neither has a cure that can completely resolve the condition.

For these reasons, people often confuse IBD with IBS. However, the two conditions are different in the following ways:

- IBD is a more severe condition that may lead to a number of complications, including malnutrition and damage to the bowel.

- IBD occurs due to an overactive immune system, which leads to inflammation throughout the gut and gastrointestinal tract. IBS usually develops due to digestive problems or an oversensitive gut.

- Treating IBD involves medications that reduce inflammation. People with IBS can reduce their symptoms by making changes to their diet or lifestyle.

Causes and risk factors

Several factors can contribute to the development of IBD. For example, it may occur because the immune system has an irregular response to bacteria, viruses, or food particles. This can trigger an inflammatory reaction in the gut.

Research has also linked Escherichia coli to Crohn's disease.

Although there is currently no single confirmed cause of IBD, there are several potential factors that can increase a person's risk of developing each of the conditions within IBD.

The sections below will discuss these in more detail.

Risk factors for ulcerative colitis

• Age: Most people receive a diagnosis at around 15–30 years of age or after 60 years of age.

• Ethnicity: People of Jewish descent seem to have a high risk of ulcerative colitis than other ethnic groups.

• Genetics: People with a close relative who has ulcerative colitis have a higher risk of developing it themselves.

Risk factors for Crohn's disease

Health professionals do not fully understand what causes Crohn's disease. However, they have identified several factors that may increase a person's risk of developing it, including:

- Genetics: People who have a parent or sibling with Crohn's disease are more likely to develop it themselves.

- Medications: The use of certain medications — including nonsteroidal anti-inflammatory medications (NSAIDs), birth control, and antibiotics — may increase the risk of Crohn's disease.

- Smoking: This habit can increase the risk of Crohn's by double.

- Diet: A diet that contains high levels of fat can also increase the risk of Crohn's disease.

Symptoms

The symptoms of IBD may vary according to the type, location, severity.

People might experience periods when symptoms worsen (flares) and periods with few or no symptoms (remission). Flares may vary in amount, intensity, and duration.

The most common symptoms are:

- Diarrhea, sometimes with blood and mucus

- Abdominal pain

- Loss of appetite and weight loss

- Unexplained fever and tiredness

- Delayed growth and maturation, particularly with Crohn's disease

Complications

Health professionals have linked a number of complications to IBD. Some of them could be life threatening.

According to the NIDDK, some possible complications of Crohn's disease include:

- bowel obstruction
- colon cancer
- fistulas, which are abnormal tunnels in the gut
- small tears in the anus, or anal fissures
- ulcers in the mouth, intestines, anus, or perineum, which is the area between the genitals and anus
- malnutrition

They also suggest that ulcerative colitis can cause the following complications:

- rectal bleeding, which may lead to iron deficiency anemia

- dehydration

- poor absorption of nutrients

- reduced bone density, possibly leading to osteopenia or osteoporosis

Diagnosis

The diagnosis of IBD may be suspected on the basis of the medical history, but the final determination depends on the results of diagnostic tests. The workup may include:

- Blood tests

- Stool infectious workup to rule out an infection and stool inflammatory marker

- X-rays

- CT or MRI scans, to detect fistulas in the small intestine or anal region

A health professional may also request endoscopic procedures. During these, they will insert a flexible probe with a camera attached through the anus.

These procedures help reveal any intestinal damage and allow the health professional to take a small sample of tissue for examination.

Some types of endoscopic procedure a health professional may use to diagnose IBD include:

- Colonoscopy: They use this to examine the entire colon.

- Flexible sigmoidoscopy: This examination helps them check the final section of the colon.

- Upper endoscopy: This procedure allows them to examine the esophagus, the stomach, and the first part of the small intestine.

Treatment

The aim of treatment is to heal the intestines and confirm this on repeat endoscopy. Even though a medical cure is not yet possible, control of symptoms and disease can be very effective in majority of patients. The number of medications available continues to increase and new treatments can be expected in the future. The most common medications used to treat IBD are:

- Antibiotics such as metronidazole and ciprofloxacin

- ASA anti-inflammatory drugs such as Asacol®, Azulfidine®, Colazol®, Pentasa®, Rowasa® and Lialda®

- Steroids, such as prednisone, prednisolone or budesonide

- Immunomodulators such as Imuran®(azathioprine), Purinethol®(6MP, and methotrexate

- Biologics, such as Remicade®, Inflectra (Biosimilar to Remicade®) Humira®, Cimzia®, Entyvio®, Stelara® and Xeljanz®

- Nutritional therapy can be used to induce and maintain remission in Crohn's disease

IBD Diet

Certain foods make IBD symptoms worse. Crafting an anti-inflammatory diet unique to your condition can help you reduce flares

Diet is important for everyone. Eating the right foods in the right quantities supplies your body with the nutrition it needs to stay healthy.

When you have inflammatory bowel disease, getting proper nutrition can be tricky. Your small intestine absorbs the nutrients from the food you eat. When you have chronic inflammation and other IBD symptoms, you may not absorb all the nutrients or digest things as well. That can lead to serious problems like malnutrition, weight loss and nutrient deficiencies.

To prevent these complications and make eating enjoyable, you need to pay close attention to what you put into your body and how your digestive system reacts.

What's in an IBD diet plan?

Crafting a diet specific to your condition, whether it's Crohn's disease, ulcerative colitis or inflammatory bowel disease that doesn't fit into either category, is complicated. The foods that trigger your Crohn's or colitis symptoms can be different than what causes problems for someone else. But there are several key ingredients to creating your own inflammatory bowel disease diet:

1. Smaller meals – Eat less, more often. Smaller meals — say six meals a day instead of a traditional breakfast, lunch and dinner — help reduce the load on your digestive tract.

2. Fluids and electrolytes – Frequent bouts of diarrhea deplete your body of water and nutrients. Drink half your body weight in ounces of water and replenish sodium, potassium and electrolytes with sports drinks.

3. Vitamins and minerals – People with Crohn's disease are at greater risk for nutrient deficiencies. Those with ulcerative colitis are more likely to be anemic. You may need to take daily multivitamins or supplements to complement a well-balanced, nutrient-rich diet.

4. Protein – While many think of vitamins and minerals, protein is also a nutrient. Eat your weight in kilograms of protein and increase your intake to restore losses after flares.

5. Higher calories – When your body has trouble processing foods, you may have to up your intake to make up for it. Eating more calories is especially important in recovering from flares and restoring lost weight.

6. Trigger food avoidance – Some things are going to make your symptoms worse. Always monitor your symptoms after eating so you can avoid those foods in the future.

What foods reduce inflammation and other symptoms of IBD?

The goals of treatment for inflammatory bowel syndrome are to improve inflammation and, ideally, get rid of it altogether. Once the inflammation is under control, the other digestive issues go away too.

You may have heard about anti-inflammatory diets or anti-inflammatory foods. A good IBD diet is a type of anti-inflammatory diet, incorporating most of the standard recommendations for a healthy diet. While you still need to create your own list of foods to eat and foods to avoid based on the triggers you and your doctors have identified, there are some general guidelines you can follow.

Foods to Include in Your IBD Diet

Your triggers will inevitably reduce your food choices. But you should still aim to eat a diverse, nutrient-dense diet to help keep your inflammatory bowel disease under control. Your diet should include a healthy mix of:

1. Fiber – Fiber can be a problematic nutrient. It's an essential part of a healthy diet, but one that commonly brings on symptoms during a flare. Focus on sources of soluble fiber (which help reduce diarrhea) like beans, fleshy fruits, oats and barley and eat other whole grains and high-fiber foods as you can tolerate.

2. Lean proteins – Too much fat can lead to poor protein absorption and make your symptoms

worse. Stick to low-fat sources of protein like chicken, turkey, fish, eggs and tofu.

3. Fruits and veggies – Eating a colorful array of plants provides a diverse mix of vitamins and minerals. If the fibrous peels and seeds cause digestive troubles, remove those before eating.

4. Calcium-rich foods – IBD, and especially Crohn's disease, can lead to lactose intolerance. So you may need to get your calcium from non-dairy sources canned fish or dark green vegetables. For your dairy fix, you can choose lactose-free or non-dairy alternatives to milk, yogurt and cheese.

5. Probiotics – Inflammatory bowel disease can flush the "good" bacteria out of your gut. Yogurt, kimchi, miso, sauerkraut, tempeh and other

sources of live bacteria can help bring your gut bacteria back into balance.

Foods to Avoid with IBD

There is no reason to avoid any food unless it triggers or worsens your symptoms. You want to get as many nutrients from as many different sources as you can. But if you haven't yet identified the foods that trigger your flares of Crohn's, ulcerative colitis or IBD, these are common culprits:

- Fatty, greasy or fried foods

- Hot or spicy foods

- Raw, high-fiber fruits and vegetables

- Nuts, seeds and beans

- Caffeinated or sugary beverages

- Alcoholic beverages

- Candy, sweets and other sources of added sugar

Alcohol, caffeine and spicy foods can irritate anyone's colon. So the problems can be worse if you have inflammatory bowel disease. Fat, sugar and fiber are all harder to digest. So you may need to stick to foods that are low in these categories or eat sources with higher contents in moderation.

What to Eat During a Crohn's or Colitis Flare

Some foods trigger cramping, bloating or diarrhea — all things you want to avoid if your inflammatory bowel disease is flaring up. When your symptoms come back, it's best to stick to the basics. Stay away from anything on the "Foods to Avoid" list that may make things worse. Instead, eat these foods plain and use boiling, grilling and steaming as your primary cooking methods:

- Vegetables: Carrots, spinach, asparagus, potatoes

- Fruits: Applesauce, canned pears or peaches, bananas, melons, avocados

- Refined grains: White rice, bread and pasta

- Proteins: Peanut butter, salmon, cooked eggs, plain chicken or turkey

Once your IBD flare-up is under control, you can slowly incorporate foods back into your normal diet, one or two at a time every few days. Start with things you know you can tolerate — liquids first, then soft solids. And slowly increase your calories, protein and fiber to return to a healthy diet that may have suffered from poor appetite or weight loss.

Whether you're in remission or in the midst of a flare, your diet is one of the keys to managing inflammatory bowel disease.

IBD DIET RECIPES

In this part are recipes to keep your IBD at bay.

Crayfish salad with rice

Preparation time

25 minutes

Ingredients

- Crayfish handful
- Rice, White for one personRice, Brown for one person
- Rice, Wild for one person
- ½ Avocado choped
- 2 Radishes chopped
- 1 Beetroot cooked, chopped
- 4 Olives chopped (optional)
- Cucumber 3cm piece, chopped

Instructions

1. Cook the rice according to the packet instructions.

2. Add the rest of the chopped salad ingredients and crayfish on top and serve.

Broccoli & kale green soup

Preparation time

35 minutes

Ingredients

- 1.200l Chicken Stock1.200l Vegetable Stock
- 2 large Broccoli heads
- 2 large Kale handfuls
- 800g Cannellini beans (2 cans)
- 4 Garlic cloves, pealed and chopped

- 2 Onions roughly chopped

- 1tbsp Olive Oil

- Salt to season

- Black pepper to season

Instructions

1. If you are vegetarian/vegan then swap the chicken stock for vegetable stock.

2. Heat the olive oil on a medium heat in a large saucepan. Add the onion and garlic and cook for 5-10 minutes until soft. Add the cumin, salt and pepper and stir through, heating for another minute or two

3. Add the stock, broccoli, kale and cannellini beans and simmer for around 15 minutes

4. Blend the soup with a hand blender (or in a food processor)

5. Season to taste and enjoy!

Note

This soup freezes well if you have any left over (or if you want to batch cook to save time at a later date).

Bouillabaisse

Preparation time

25 minutes

Ingredients

- 5 Garlic cloves
- 2tsp Olive Oil
- ½tsp Fennel seed
- 2 Bay Leaves
- 3tsp Tomato Puree
- Sea Salt to taste
- ½ Fennel bulb
- 200g Tomatoes tinned
- 5cup Fish Stock
- Prawns large handful
- Mussels large handful
- Cod large handful
- Monkfish large handful

Instructions

1. Put the olive oil into a pan and heat. Add the garlic, fennel seeds and fennel bulb and cook for a few minutes, making sure they don't burn

2. Add tomato puree and cook for ½ minute with the chopped tomatoes

3. Add the bay leaves and fish stock and cook for 15 mins

4. Add the monk fish and cook for 2 - 3 mins

5. Then add the chopped cod and mussels. When the mussels start to open, add the prawns and adjust the seasoning

Roasted root vegetable soup

Preparation time

75 minutes

Ingredients

1. 50ml Olive Oil

2. 1 small Butternut Squash peeled, seeded, chopped

3. 2 Carrots chopped

4. 1 large Parsnips chopped

5. 1 small Swede chopped

6. 2 Leeks chopped (optional)

7. 1 Onion chopped

8. 3 Bay Leaves

9. 4 Thyme sprigs

10. 3 Rosemary sprigs

11. 1.200l Vegetable Stock

12. Salt

13. Black pepper

Instructions

1. You can mix and match the vegetables to create a soup you can eat.

2. Preheat the oven to 200C (400F)

3. Add the chopped vegetables to a large bowl and coat them in the olive oil. Spread them out

over a large baking tray (or two is necessary) so that they in a single layer

4. Add the bay, thyme and rosemary in amongst the vegetables

5. Roast for around 50 minutes, unless they are soft. You should turn the vegetables a few times during cooking

6. Take out from the oven and remove the herbs. Transfer the vegetables to a large saucepan

7. Add the vegetable stock and bring to the boil then reduce the heat and simmer for 10 minutes. Season with salt and pepper

8. Blend the vegetables using a food processor or blender until smooth

9. Reheat the soup before serving

10. If you have any left over you can freeze it in individual portions

Blueberry protein smoothie bowl

Preparation time

5 minutes

Ingredients

- 1scoop Whey Protein Powder (Strawberry)

- 1 Bananas frozen
- 200ml Almond Milk
- 1tbsp Frozen Fruits
- 2tsp Choc Shot (liquid chocolate)
- 1tsp Bee Pollen

Instructions

1. Add all ingredients into a blender except choc shot, bee pollen mixed seeds

2. Once the blended ingredients is at a desired consistency swirl the choc shot into the mixture

3. Top with bee pollen & mixed seeds (optional)

Quick no-tomato sauce

Preparation time

60 minutes

Ingredients

- 1 small Onion

- 4 Garlic cloves

- 125g Carrots

- 2 medium Sweet Potatoes

- 3tbsp Lemon Juice

- 1tbsp Balsamic Vinegar

- Salt to taste

- Black pepper (to taste)

- 1 large Beetroot cooked

- Water

- 1tbsp Olive Oil

Instructions

Roughly chop all the vegetables, including the onion and garlic

Heat 1 tbsp of olive oil in a saucepan and add the onion and garlic. Cook until soft then add the carrots and sweet potato and cook for a couple of minutes

Add all the other ingredients, except for the cooked beetroot

Add water to just cover the vegetables and bring to the boil

1. Reduce the heat and cover.

2. Simmer for around 30-45 minutes until the carrots and sweet potato are completely soft

3. Transfer the mixture to a food processor and add the beetroot.

4. Blend until smooth. You may need to do this in a couple of batches.

5. If the sauce is too thick you can add a little water

6. Your sauce is now ready to be used in the same way as chopped tomatoes or tomato passata in pasta dishes.

7. It makes quite a few servings so if you aren't going to use it all up within a few days then you can freeze it.

8. Just divide it into freezable containers or bags in individual portions.

Chicken salad with sweet potato mash

Preparation time

30 minutes

Ingredients

- 1 medium Sweet Potato

- Chicken cooked

- Radishes

- Cucumber

- Avocados

- Beetroot cooked

Instructions

1. Peel and roughly chop the sweet potato.

2. Add it to a pan of boiling water and cook for around 15 minutes, or until the potato is soft

3. Drain and mash the potato

4. Chop your salad. You can use whatever ratio of salad ingredients you like (and whatever salad you can eat)

5. Serve the salad and potato with the chicken

Prawn and chorizo paella

Preparation time

55 minutes

Ingredients

2tbsp Olive Oil2tbsp Coconut Oil

100g Paella Rice

½ Onion

350ml Chicken Stock (or fish, veg stock)

1tsp Turmeric

1tsp Paprika smoked

2tbsp Lemon Juice2tbsp Lime Juice

5 Saffron pieces (optional)

30g Chorizo (ensure gluten & dairy free)

100g Prawns large

Instructions

1. Slice the onion and garlic and fry them in the olive oil over a medium heat until they are soft.

2. Pour the rice into the pan and stir around so that it is coated in the olive oil.

3. Once coated add half the stock.

4. Add the paprika, saffron and turmeric to the mixture and also a tablespoon of the lemon or lime juice.

5. Season with salt and pepper and bring to the boil and then leave to simmer, stirring

occasionally to prevent the mixture from sticking to the bottom of the pan.

6. Meanwhile, chop the chorizo into small chunks (or big ones if you prefer!) and add to the pan.

7. After 10 minutes add any vegetables (see below) and stir them through the rice.

8. As the rice absorbs the stock add more to the mixture.

9. Once all the liquid has been absorbed by the rice (this may take 20-30 minutes) taste it to check if the rice is cooked.

10. If it is still hard or too crunchy for your taste then add a bit of water and continue to boil.

11. Repeat this process until you have rice cooked to your taste.

12. Add the prawns and the rest of the lemon or lime juice and cook for another 3-4minutes until the prawns are heated through.

13. Serve on its own or with a salad, garlic bread or other tapas dishes.

Note

Veg you could add: Peas, green beans, soya beans"¦..

If you don't like prawns, or just want a variation, why not add some chicken instead (or as well)?

Coronation chicken with rice

Preparation time

30 minutes

Ingredients

- 2 Chicken breasts

- Rice, White (enough for 2 people)Rice, Wild (enough for 2 people)Rice, Brown (enough for 2 people)

- 4tbsp Mayonnaise

- 4tbsp Apricot Jam

- 1tbsp Curry Powder , Mild

- 1 Carrots (Optional)

- ¼ Courgette (Zucchini) (Optional)

- 6 Mushrooms (Optional)

- Broccoli , Handful (Optional)

- Raisins , Handful (Optional)

- 1tbsp Coconut Oil 1tbsp Olive Oil

Instructions

This coronation chicken recipe deviates from a classic recipe with the inclusion of lots of vegetables. If you want to stick to a traditional coronation chicken you can leave the vegetables out. You can also use any cooking oil, I just prefer to use coconut oil.

If you don't eat meat then you can leave out the chicken and add more vegetables.

1. Cut the chicken breasts into bitesize pieces

2. Heat the coconut oil in a pan on a medium heat and add the chicken to the pan.

3. Allow to cook for 5 minutes, stirring to ensure all size of the chicken are cooking evenly.

4. If using, add the carrot at this point and cook for a few minutes and then add the other vegetables.

5. In a small bowl mix together the mayonnaise, jam and curry powder and then add to the chicken.

6. Stir the sauce in thoroughly.

7. Add the raisins (if using).

8. Allow the mixture to cook for 10-15 minutes until the chicken has cooked all the way through and the vegetables are soft.

9. Cook the rice according to the instructions on the packet.

10. Once the chicken and rice are ready serve.

Gluten free tabbouleh

Preparation time

30 minutes

Ingredients

- 100g Quinoa

- Chives chopped, handful

- Mint leaves chopped, handful

- Parsley chopped, handful

- 2tbsp Olive Oil

- 2tbsp Lemon Juice

Instructions

1. Cook the quinoa according to the pack instructions

2. Once cooked stir in the lemon juice and the herbs.

3. Season with salt and pepper

4. Serve cold with falafel, cooked chicken or as a side dish at a barbecue

Courgetti

Preparation time

30 minutes

Ingredients

- 2 medium Courgettes (Zucchini)

Instructions

1. To make courgetti you will need a spiraliser

2. To get the best courgetti you should buy courgettes that are straight and thick.

3. Start by cutting the ends off the courgettes and, if they are long, cut them in half.

4. Put your courgette into the spiraliser and follow the manufacturer's instructions to create.

5. Use courgetti in place of spaghetti or other types of pasta.

Fish or veggie cakes

Preparation time

65 minutes

Ingredients

- 3 Tuna tins (in water)3 Salmon tins (in water)3 Cannellini beans tins (in water) (vegetarian)
- 4 large Potatoes, White4 large Sweet Potatoes (Nightshade free)
- 2 large Chicken Eggs
- Gluten Free Flour HandfulPlain Flour (no longer gluten free recipe)
- Parsley Handful
- Black pepper
- Dill Handful
- Gluten free breadcrumbsBreadcrumbs (no longer gluten free recipe)

Instructions

1. Preheat the oven to 180C

2. Boil the potatoes until they're cooked but still firm enough to mash rather than mush.

3. Drain and mash thoroughly.

4. Mix in the drained tinned fish.

5. Add parsley, dill and black pepper to taste.

6. Allow mix to cool and then roll into fist sized patties.

7. Lay out three bowls - one with the flour, one with the eggs (beaten) and one with the breadcrumbs.

8. One by one, dip each of the patties in the flour then the eggs then the breadcrumbs, ensuring they're thoroughly coated in each. This will get messy!

9. Place on a baking tray, bake for 45mins and eat hot.

Leeks, sprouts and broccoli with lemon herb sauce

Preparation time

15 minutes

Ingredients

- 1 Leeks sliced
- 80g Brussels Sprouts sliced
- 80g Broccoli florets
- 20g Dairy Free Spread20g Butter

- 1tsp Parsley chopped

- Lemon Juice from quarter lemon

- Lemon Rind from half lemon

- Black pepper to taste

Instructions

1. Steam the vegetables until they have softened but still have a little 'bite'

2. Add the spread (or butter) to a small saucepan along with the parsley, lemon juice and rind.

3. Add the vegetables and heat over a medium heat until the spread has melted

4. Add some black pepper, stir the vegetables to ensure they are fully coated in the sauce and then serve.

Easy chicken basquaise

Preparation time

65 minutes

Ingredients

- 8 Chicken legs or thighs
- 4tbsp Gluten Free Flour4tbsp Plain Flour (not gluten free)
- Salt
- Black pepper
- 4tbsp Olive Oil
- 1 medium Onion
- 2 Red Peppers (Capsicum) (Optional)
- 2 Garlic cloves
- 150g Chorizo (ensure gluten & dairy free)
- 200g Arborio Rice200g Long Grain Rice
- 450ml Chicken Stock
- ½tsp Thyme Dried or fresh

- 125g Jamon Serrano (Spanish ham)
- 12 Black Olives
- 2tbsp Parsley fresh, chopped
- Courgettes (Zucchini) Half (Optional)

Instructions

1. Preheat the oven to 190c

2. Heat half the oil over a medium heat in a heavy-based pan or casserole dish.

3. Dice the onion and crush the garlic and add to the pan.

4. Cook until the onion in golden

5. Add the chorizo and vegetables and cook for a couple of minutes

6. Add the rice and stir so it is coated in the oil.

7. Add the stock, the thyme, salt and pepper and stir thoroughly.

8. Cover and cook over a low heat for 45 minutes, stirring occasionally and adding a bit of water if it becomes dry

9. Meanwhile dry the chicken using kitchen roll.

10. Put the flour in a polythene bag along with some salt and black pepper

11. . Add the chicken, seal the bag and shake until the chicken is all coated

12. Heat a frying pan over a medium heat and add the rest of the olive oil to the pan.

13. Add the chicken and cook, turning regularly, so that the flour on the outside starts to turn crispy.

14. Transfer the chicken to an oven proof dish and place in the oven for 20-30 minutes.

15. When it's cooked the juices should run clear if a knife is inserted into the centre

16. After the rice has been cooking for 45 minutes add the ham, black olives and chopped parsley.

17. Stir and cook for another 5 minutes.

18. When both the chicken and rice are cooked serve immediately.

Sweet potato chips

Preparation time

55 minutes

Ingredients

- 1 large Sweet Potato
- 1tbsp Olive Oil
- Sea Salt to season
- Black pepper to season

Instructions

1. Preheat the oven to 200C

2. Chop the sweet potato into chip sized pieces (around 1cm thick)

3. Place in a pan of boiling water for around 5 minutes then transfer to a oven proof dish (big enough that the chips are only on one layer) and sprinkle the oil over and season with salt and pepper and mix to cover

4. Place in the oven and cook for around 35 minutes, turning occasionally

5. Serve hot

Lemon cake bars

Preparation time

55 minutes

Ingredients

- 1¾ cup Gluten Free Flour
- ½ cup Icing Sugar + more for dusting
- 1 large Lemon Rind
- 9 tbsp Dairy Free Spread
- 4 large Chicken Eggs
- 1 cup Sugar, Granulated
- ¾ tsp Baking Powder
- Lemon Juice (Juice of 4 lemons)

Instructions

1. Preheat the oven to 180°C.

2. Grease an 8-inch square baking tray

3. Starting with the crust.

4. In a bowl, blend a cup of the flour (around 150g), all the icing sugar and lemon zest.

5. Break up any clumps of lemon zest.

6. Add the spread and mix with a fork until well-combined.

7. Press the mixture into the bottom of the baking tray.

8. Place it in the centre of the preheated oven and bake for about 15 minutes until firm

9. Remove from the oven and allow to cool briefly

10. Now make the custard layer.

11. In a medium-sized bowl, place the eggs, granulated sugar, baking powder, lemon juice and remaining 2/3 cup flour, whisking to combine

12. Pour the custard mixture onto the baked crust and return to the oven until it's set (20 to 25 minutes).

13. The custard is set when it doesn't wobble when the tray is shaken. Remove it from the oven and allow to cool for about 20 minutes

14. Place in the fridge to chill until firm, ideally overnight.

15. Remove from the tray and slice into bars.

16. Lightly dust with icing sugar

High protein breakfast pancakes

Preparation time

8 minutes

Ingredients

- 1 medium Chicken Egg
- 1 Bananas Mashed
- 1tsp Coconut Oil
- 1tsp Honey
- 1scoop Whey Protein Powder (Vanilla)

Instructions

Pancakes are one of the most versatile dishes in the world!

For this recipe I have kept it simple and used a vanilla whey protein powder & bananas

You can substitute the honey for a sweetener if your prefer and for a grain free recipe simply remove the muesli or add nuts and seeds.

1. Mix 1 banana with 1 egg until smooth.

2. Slowly add the protein powder smoothing out any lumps as they appear

3. To recreate this stack use a mini frying pan or put 2-3 dollops in a larger pan for quicker results.

4. Layered each pancake with chopped banana, a drizzle of honey and scatter the top with muesli.

Smoked salmon frittata

Preparation time

20 minutes

Ingredients

1. 2 Chicken Eggs

2. Sweet Potatoes handful, roasted

3. Courgettes (Zucchini) handful, roasted

4. Spinach handful, wilted

5. 50g Smoked Salmon

6. 1tsp Dill chopped

7. Salt to season

8. Black pepper to season

9. 1tsp Olive Oil

Instructions

1. Turn the grill on to a medium heat

2. Place the olive oil in a small frying pan on the hob over a medium heat

3. Add the roasted sweet potato, courgette, and spinach to heat up for a few minutes, stirring occasionally

4. Crack the eggs into a bowl, season with salt and pepper and whisk with a fork until combined

5. Tear the smoked salmon into pieces and place evenly on top of the vegetables, then pour over the eggs

6. Allow the frittata to cook for 5 minutes or so until it starts to harden and finish cooking the top under the grill for a few minutes

7. Sprinkle with dill before serving

Note

If you want to make a large frittata to serve more or have for lunches over several days then use a large frying pan and triple the ingredient quantities.

Milk kefir recipe

Preparation time

10 minutes

Ingredients

- 1cup Milk whole (full fat)
- 1tsp Milk kefir grains

Instructions

1. Picture above shows activated milk kefir grains.

2. Pour the milk into a glass contained such as a jar or drinking glass

3. Stir in the kefir grains

4. Cover with a cheese cloth, paper towel, muslin or napkin and secure with an elastic band

5. Leave at room temperature for 12 to 24 hours (the ideal temperature is 21c and takes around 24 hours at this temperature, on hotter days it will take less and will take longer on colder days).

6. Once it has thickened and tastes tangy it is ready. It it has been 48 hours and the mixture hasn't thickened then strain out the kefir grains and try again.

7. Strain

8. You can then use the grains to make a new batch of kefir.

9. They should be able to continue making kefir every 24 hours.

10. If you are not going to make another batch straight away then transfer the grains into a cup of milk and store in the fridge (for up to a month), otherwise return back to step 1 of this recipe.

11. Enjoy! The kefir can be kept in the fridge for up to a week.

Notes

The grains will multiply over time so you may which to discard the old ones as new ones appear or you could pass them onto a friend to make kefir themselves.

The grains do not like metal so minimise the time they have in contact with metal (such as teaspoons, strainer) and always use glass to culture the grains in.

Swede chips

Preparation time

55 minutes

Ingredients

- 1 Swede

- 1tbsp Olive Oil

- 2tbsp Soy Sauce (not gluten free)2tbsp Tamari (use this for gluten free)
- 1tbsp Paprika smoked

Instructions

1. Preheat the oven to 200C

2. Trim the swede and chop into chip sized pieces (around 1cm thick)

3. Place in a pan of boiling water for around 5 minutes then transfer to a oven proof dish (big enough that the chips are only on one layer) and sprinkle the oil, soy sauce (or tamari) and paprika over the swede and mix to cover

4. Place in the oven and cook for around 35 minutes, turning occasionally

5. Serve hot

Easy Japanese 'sushi' handrolls

Preparation time

30 minutes

Ingredients

- 1 Sushi Nori packet
- 5tbsp Mayonnaise
- 1 Avocado (Optional)
- 250g Smoked Salmon
- 1 Carrots (Optional)
- 4 Radishes (Optional)

- ½tsp Wasabi (Optional)
- Sushi Rice prepared to serve 2Rice, White for 2 people

Instructions

1. Cook the rice according to the instructions on the packet.

2. While the rice is cooking prepare the carrot, avocado and radish by cutting into long, thin strips.

3. Mix together the mayonnaise and wasabi (if you are using)

4. Once the rice is cooked allow to cool a little before starting to make your handrolls (or if you have time allow to cool completely).

5. Take a sheet of nori and cut it in half.

6. Spread a little mayonnaise onto the sheet diagonally from the top left corner to the middle bottom.

7. On top of that add a strip of rice, followed by a piece of smoked salmon and on top your vegetables.

8. Roll the nori into a cone shape and enjoy.

9. If you like wasabi then you can add more to your mayonnaise.

10. You can use any combination of vegetables and meat/fish in these rolls.

Beef or veggie lentil dhal

Preparation time

55 minutes

Ingredients

- 2tbsp Coconut Oil2tbsp Olive Oil
- ½ Onion (optional)
- 3 Garlic Cloves
- 250g Beef steak (optional)250g Lamb diced (optional)
- 1 Carrots
- 2tsp Cumin ground
- Ginger fresh, 2.5cm piece
- 2tsp Turmeric ground
- 1tsp Chili Powder mild (optional)

- 1tsp Garam Masala

- 225g Lentils, Red

- 400ml Water

- 400ml Coconut Milk

- Lime Juice from 2 limes

- 4tbsp Coriander fresh

- Sea Salt (to season)

- Black pepper (to season)

- 25g Almonds flakes (optional)

Instructions

1. Heat the oil in a heavy-based saucepan.

2. Add the onion and cook for a few minutes until soft. While it is cooking crush the garlic, chop the carrots into thin slices and, if using, cut the beef into bite-sized chunks

3. Add the garlic and carrot and cook for another few minutes.

4. At this stage you can also add any other chopped vegetables you like (such as courgette, green beans, broccoli).

5. Meanwhile use a fine grater to grate the ginger

6. Add the ginger and spices (cumin, turmeric, chilli powder, garam masala) to the pan and stir thoroughly, cooking for a minute

7. If using beef at it now and cook for a couple of minutes, stirring to cover in the spices

8. Add the lentils, water, coconut milk and season and with salt and pepper.

9. Bring to the boil then reduce the heat and cover the pan.

10. Simmer for around 35 minutes, stirring regularly to prevent the lentils from sticking to the bottom of the pan. If the mixture becomes dry add a little water

11. While the dhal is cooking toast the almonds (if using).

12. To do this heat a dry frying pan.

13. Once it is hot add the almonds to the pan and cook for a few minutes, stirring very regularly to prevent them from burning.

14. Remove from the heat and put aside

15. After 35 minutes add the lime juice and fresh coriander and season again with salt and pepper if needed.

16. Leave to cook for another 10 minutes

17. Once ready serve in bowls and sprinkle over the toasted almonds and some fresh coriander

Lemongrass steamed sea bass

Preparation time

25 minutes

Ingredients

- 2 Sea Bass fillets
- 1tbsp Olive Oil
- 2 Garlic Cloves
- 1 Lemongrass Stalk1tbsp Lemongrass Paste
- 1tsp Thyme , Fresh
- 1tsp Coriander , Fresh
- 1tbsp Tamari1tbsp Soy Sauce (not gluten free)
- 1tsp Sesame Oil
- 1tsp Chili Flakes (Optional) (Not nightshade free)

Instructions

1. Boil a saucepan of water

2. Chop the garlic, lemongrass, coriander and thyme.

3. Mix them together with the olive oil and then rub the mixture into the sea bass fillets

4. Place the fillets into two square pieces of baking paper and place the sea bass fillets in the centre of each piece.

5. You now want to enclose the fish in the paper, leaving some air inside to steam the fish.

6. Fold both of the longest sides of the paper into the middle and then twist the paper at either end of the fish so that you have something that looks a bit like a Christmas cracker

7. Place a large sieve or colander over the pan of boiling water and place the fish parcels inside.

8. They should now sit above the water.

9. Leave for around 5 minutes.

10. When the fish is cooked it should have all turned white (be careful when opening the parcels as hot air will escape)

11. Mix together the tamari (or soy sauce), sesame oil and chilli flakes (if using).

12. Pour over the fish

13. Serve with rice noodles, plain rice, stir fired veg, stir fried green veg and/or sesame samphire.

Nightshade free guacamole

Preparation time

5 minutes

Ingredients

1. 1 Avocado

2. 1 Lime Juice

3. Coriander Fresh, Handful

4. ½tbsp Olive Oil

5. Sea Salt , to taste

6. Black pepper , to taste

Instructions

1. Add all the ingredients into a blender and blitz together until the avocado has been completely blended.

Zesty summer salad

Preparation time

10 minutes

Ingredients

- ½ large Apple grated

- 2 small Carrots grated

- 1 medium Courgette (Zucchini) grated

- ¼ Lemon juice only

- 1tbsp Yoghurt - Plain
- ½tbsp Mayonnaise
- ¼tbsp Honey
- Sesame Seeds (optional) for sprinkling

Instructions

1. Mix together the grated apple, carrots, courgette and lemon juice in a bowl

2. Separately mix together the yogurt, mayonnaise and honey

3. Combine the two, stirring well

4. Sprinkle the sesame seeds (if using) on top

Chicken wrapped in bacon with pineapple and roasted vegetables

Preparation time

55 minutes

Ingredients

- 2 Chicken Breasts
- 4 Bacon rashers
- 2 Pineapples rings
- 1 large Carrots
- 1 large Parsnips
- 1 medium Sweet Potato
- 2tbsp Coconut Oil2tbsp Olive Oil

Instructions

1. Preheat the oven to 200c

2. Chop the vegetables into batons (peeling their skins if you can't tolerate them).

3. Then place the veg into a roasting tray and add the coconut oil (you can use olive oil instead if you don't like the taste of coconut oil).

4. Place into the oven for 30-40mins.

5. Remove to stir regularly ensuring the vegetables are coated in the coconut oil as it melts in the oven.

6. When they are cooked they should be golden and soft

7. Place a pineapple ring on top of each chicken breast and then wrap 2 pieces of bacon over the top of each breast, tucking the ends of the bacon underneath the chicken.

8. Place on a second baking tray and put into the oven after the vegetables have been cooking for around 10-15 minutes

9. After the chicken has been in the oven for around 20-30 minutes check to see if it's cooked. If it's done the juices should run clear when you insert a knife into the centre of the chicken. If in doubt you should cut the chicken breast to check. The time it takes to cook can vary depending on the size of the chicken breast and your oven.

10. If it is still pink/bloody inside then leave it for another 5 minutes and check again

11. Once ready, remove the chicken and vegetables from the oven and serve

Gluten free teriyaki sauce

Preparation time

45 minutes

Ingredients

- 150ml Tamari

- 150ml Mirin

- 50ml Sake50ml Shaoxing rice wine ensure gluten free

- 50g Sugar

Instructions

1. Place all of the ingredients in a saucepan and bring to the boil then reduce the heat so the sauce is simmering

2. Leave to simmer for around 15 minutes. It should reduce by around a third

3. Remove from the heat and leave to cool. As it cools it should become like a syrup

4. Pour into a bottle and keep in the fridge for up to a month

5. Use it on salmon, chicken or vegetables

Bacon, eggs and avocado

Preparation time

10 minutes

Ingredients

- 3 Bacon rashers, choose organic

- 2 medium Chicken Eggs

- ½ Avocado sliced

Instructions

1. Heat a frying pan and add the bacon.

2. Cook for around 5 minutes or until the bacon is cooked to your taste.

3. Meanwhile add a little oil to a new frying pan and heat, or to half of the pan with the bacon in it, and crack in the eggs.

4. Cook until the while of the egg is cooked through

Gluten free teriyaki sauce

Preparation time

45 minutes

Ingredients

- 150ml Tamari
- 150ml Mirin

- 50ml Sake50ml Shaoxing rice wine ensure gluten free
- 50g Sugar

Instructions

1. Place all of the ingredients in a saucepan and bring to the boil then reduce the heat so the sauce is simmering.

2. Leave to simmer for around 15 minutes. It should reduce by around a third

3. Remove from the heat and leave to cool.

4. As it cools it should become like a syrup

5. Pour into a bottle and keep in the fridge for up to a month

6. Use it on salmon, chicken or vegetables

Egg fried rice

Preparation time

25 minutes

Ingredients

- Rice, White for 2 peopleRice, Brown for 2 people

- Rice, Wild for 2 people

- 2 Chicken Eggs

- ½ Chorizo ring, optional (check for gluten and dairy free)

- Broccoli handful, chopped

- Courgettes (Zucchini) handful, chopped

- Sea Salt to season

- Black pepper to season

- 2tbsp Tamari

- 2tbsp Soy Sauce (no longer gluten free recipe)

- Spring Onions (optional)

- 2tsp Sesame Oil2tsp Olive Oil

- 1 small Carrot shredded

Instructions

1. Cook the rice according to the packet instructions, drain and put aside to cool

2. Chop whatever vegetables/meat you are using into small pieces. The ones for the recipe are just a suggestion - you can add whatever veggies and meat you like....such as cooked chicken, ham, sweetcorn, peas, beans, peppers

3. Heat a wok or large frying pan and add the oil to the pan. Then add the meat and vegetables and stir fry until they start to soften a little. Then move the mixture to one side and crack the eggs into the empty side of the pan. Mix the eggs together and then allow to cook for a minute. Before they are fully cooked mix the eggs together with the meat/vegetables so that they are scrambled among everything else

4. Add the tamari, salt and pepper and mix thoroughly. Heat for a couple of minutes and then serve

Easy chicken basquaise

Preparation time

65 minutes

Ingredients

- 8 Chicken legs or thighs

- 4tbsp Gluten Free Flour4tbsp Plain Flour (not gluten free)

- Salt

- Black pepper

- 4tbsp Olive Oil
- 1 medium Onion
- 2 Red Peppers (Capsicum) (Optional)
- 2 Garlic cloves
- 150g Chorizo (ensure gluten & dairy free)
- 200g Arborio Rice200g Long Grain Rice
- 450ml Chicken Stock
- ½tsp Thyme Dried or fresh
- 125g Jamon Serrano (Spanish ham)
- 12 Black Olives
- 2tbsp Parsley fresh, chopped
- Courgettes (Zucchini) Half (Optional)

Instructions

1. Preheat the oven to 190c

2. Heat half the oil over a medium heat in a heavy-based pan or casserole dish.

3. Dice the onion and crush the garlic and add to the pan.

4. Cook until the onion in golden

5. Add the chorizo and vegetables and cook for a couple of minutes

6. Add the rice and stir so it is coated in the oil.

7. Add the stock, the thyme, salt and pepper and stir thoroughly.

8. Cover and cook over a low heat for 45 minutes, stirring occasionally and adding a bit of water if it becomes dry

9. Meanwhile dry the chicken using kitchen roll.

10. Put the flour in a polythene bag along with some salt and black pepper.

11. Add the chicken, seal the bag and shake until the chicken is all coated

12. Heat a frying pan over a medium heat and add the rest of the olive oil to the pan.

13. Add the chicken and cook, turning regularly, so that the flour on the outside starts to turn crispy.

14. Transfer the chicken to an oven proof dish and place in the oven for 20-30 minutes.

15. When it's cooked the juices should run clear if a knife is inserted into the centre

16. After the rice has been cooking for 45 minutes add the ham, black olives and chopped parsley.

17. Stir and cook for another 5 minutes

18. When both the chicken and rice are cooked serve immediately

Turkey and spinach meatball

Preparation time

50 minutes

ingredients:

- 1 lb. ground turkey

- 2 eggs

- 1/3 c. water

- 1/2 c. grated Parmesan cheese

- 1 c. gluten-free breadcrumbs (or regular if you are not gluten-free)

- 1/4 c. packed frozen spinach, thawed

- 1 tsp. onion powder

- 1 1/2 tsp. garlic powder

- 1 tsp. dried oregano

- 1 tsp. salt

- 1 tsp. pepper

Instructions

1. Mix all ingredients in a large bowl.

2. Roll into 2-inch balls, and evenly place on a non-stick baking pan

3. Bake on 350F for 30 minutes

4. You can freeze them for up to 1 month.

5. Sign up for emails

6. Enter email address